Published in the United Kingdom by Roby Education Ltd., 3, Lyndhurst, Maghull, Merseyside L31 6DY
for The Joint Epilepsy Council of the UK and Ireland (JEC) and the International Bureau for Epilepsy (IBE)
with the aid of generous financial support from Hoechst Marion Roussel

The Illustrated Encyclopaedia of Epilepsy
1st edition 1997
ISBN 0 948270 65 9

Printed in the United Kingdom by Alden Colour, Oxford.

Acknowledgements:
Paula Cant, Viv Chadwick, Gerald Chew, Judy Cochrane, Bijel Desai, Geraldine Dunne, Karl Drewek,
Jay Henderson, Lisa Henry, Phil Jones, Liedewij Jepsen, Julian Knowles, Philip Lee, Sue Macdonald,
Tony Marson, David Nodder, Shishir Patel, Sally Phipps, Anita Rogan, Colette Rogan, Joe Russell,
Heather Trappe, Paul Skelley, Caroline Turnbull, Ben White, Mandy Williams.

Photographic Sources:
James Cant, Philip Coppell, The Image Bank, Manchester (posed by models), Oxford Instruments Ltd
(Medilog®), Medelec Ltd., Nicolet Biomedical Ltd., Picker International Ltd., Science Photo Library.

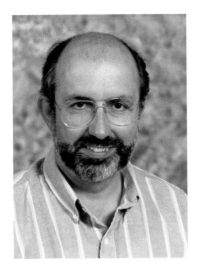

Because epilepsy is the most common of all neurological disorders it is not surprising that the special epilepsy clinics I hold in Liverpool are busy. Ideally I would like to be able to spend more time with patients to explain more about their epilepsy but, because of the demands, this is not always possible.

I was delighted, therefore, to be asked to edit this Encyclopaedia of Epilepsy because I believe that the more people know about their epilepsy the better. This book is a step forward in epilepsy education, not only for those who have the condition but also for their friends, relations and workmates. It comes as a successor to the "The Illustrated Junior Encyclopaedia of Epilepsy", first published in 1995. I hope that it will be as successful as that book in achieving a wider knowledge of epilepsy in the community.

The text is illustrated throughout with photographs and is cross referenced so that individual areas of interest can be followed through in logical sequence. The entries dealing with the voluntary sector organisations are, I hope, useful. These organisations work tirelessly in helping people with epilepsy and their worth should not be underestimated when it comes to the overall management and treatment of epilepsy. Take note of their telephone numbers and their addresses. They could be as useful to you as they undoubtedly are to me.

My thanks are offered to the Joint Epilepsy Council of the UK and Ireland (JEC) and the International Bureau for Epilepsy (IBE) for inviting me to be associated with this Encyclopaedia.

Thanks are also offered for the sponsorship by Hoechst Marion Roussel which made publication possible.

David Chadwick

Professor of Neurology, University of Liverpool

Absence Seizure (Atypical) These absence seizures occur across the whole age range with people who have some form of brain damage. The seizures last longer than simple absence seizures and result in massive jerks or a very sudden loss of muscle tone - either of which can cause the person to fall to the ground with some force. They may injure themselves in the process and many have to wear protective headgear to avoid head injuries.

Absence Seizure (Typical) These types of generalised seizures are sometimes referred to as "petit mal" seizures. The condition always begins in childhood and is relatively rare, accounting for 4% of childhood epilepsy. It is more common in girls than in boys. Simple absence seizures occur suddenly, provoking a brief trance-like state. Affected children stare blankly ahead or into space and their failure to respond when spoken to can mean that they get into trouble in school for not paying attention. There are serious educational implications for children whose absence seizures have not been recognised and treated. Once the condition has been diagnosed it is treated with antiepileptic drugs and in many cases the children affected become seizure free and enjoy a normal education. In the majority of cases medication can be safely discontinued in adulthood when the condition usually ceases. Up to one third of children who experience absence seizures may, however, have waking tonic clonic seizures in later life.

ACTH Adrenocorticotrophic hormone. This may be helpful in treatment of infantile spasms.

Adult onset seizures Seizures which begin in adulthood.

Adversive seizures Partial seizures which mainly affect the head, eyes and arms. The first stage of the seizure results in the head and the eyes being drawn to one side. A hand or an arm may become stiff and drawn upwards. This may or may not be followed by a second stage where the head, arm or leg will jerk. Following an adversive seizure some people experience a short-term one sided weakness. This is known as Todd's Paralysis.

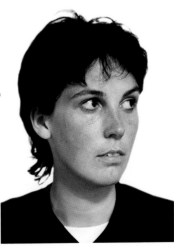

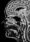

Aetiology of epilepsy

This term refers to the causes of epilepsy. In some cases a definite cause is found and the epilepsy is then referred to as symptomatic. When no definite cause is found the epilepsy is referred to as idiopathic.

Alcohol & Epilepsy

Alcohol can be the cause of seizures. 20% of alcohol dependent men and 10% of alcohol dependent women over the age of 25 develop tonic clonic seizures; the peak incidence occurring between the ages of 45 and 50 years. In some people the seizures occur 12-48 hours after a prolonged bout of drinking - so called "rum seizures". More commonly, seizures occur on alcohol withdrawal. Hospital tests seldom reveal any abnormality of the brain in these people and it is assumed that the seizures occur as a result of the direct toxic effects of the alcohol. Seizures may be the result of sudden withdrawal of alcohol or other addictive substances, a condition similar to delirium tremens (DTs). The withdrawal of a barbiturate drug such as phenobarbitone can have the same effect. "Rum seizures" are likely to disappear completely if the alcohol dependent person succeeds in giving up drinking.

In some alcohol dependent people (about 10%) the seizures are not caused directly by alcohol, but by brain damage that has resulted from head injuries sustained while under the influence of alcohol.

Most doctors advise people with epilepsy to be very cautious of drinking alcohol because the effectiveness of antiepileptic drugs can be impaired. However, there is no evidence that an occasional social drink is in any way harmful.

Ambulatory EEG monitoring

Sometimes it can be very useful to record EEGs for a lengthy period of time (sometimes in excess of a day) using portable recording equipment. Eight electrodes are fixed to the scalp and attached to a cassette recorder which can be carried around the waist. The electrical activity of the brain is recorded directly over the prescribed

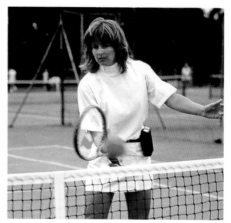

The ambulatory E.E.G. is worn on the waist. Electrodes are attached to the scalp and, in the example shown here, kept in place by a collar.

period of time. The cassette tape is fed into a computer to be read by a neurophysiologist who reports the finding back to the neurologist who is treating the person.

Anticonvulsant drug   A drug used to control epileptic seizures of a convulsive type.

Antiepileptic drug   A drug prescribed to control epileptic seizures of any type.

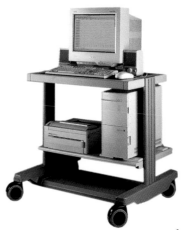

Typical computer equipment for analysing ambulatory E.E.G. recording.

Astatic Seizures   See Drop Attacks or Atonic seizures.

Ataxia   This is simply a word which means loss of co-ordination. It is sometimes caused by antiepileptic drugs, when either too large a dose is given or too many drugs are being taken. When the drug levels are monitored and the dosage corrected, people return to having their normal levels of co-ordination.

Atonic Seizures   In these types of seizure, muscle tone is lost causing the person to collapse to the ground. Sometimes referred to as "Drop Attacks" or astatic seizures, these seizures can be quite dramatic. The person falls heavily and although recovery is swift the result is often head or facial injury. The wearing of protective helmets can limit the extent of injury.

Aura   This word is applied to the signals which warn of the onset of a seizure, though, in fact, an aura is itself a simple partial seizure. Some people

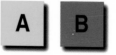

always have an aura before a longer seizure occurs. This is particularly so prior to a complex partial seizure.

Auras can take many forms. For example, one can become aware of a funny feeling in the stomach which rises into the throat. There may be a feeling of "looking in on oneself" or the sensation of a strange taste or smell; a familiar piece of music or a non existent noise may be heard. One very strange and common aura is that feeling known popularly as 'déja vu'.

A description of an aura, no matter how sketchy, is a great help to a neurologist in arriving at a correct diagnosis of the type of epilepsy and consequently prescribing the correct medication.

Automatisms

These are semi-purposeful movements usually lasting for a few minutes, which are commonly a feature of complex partial seizures. Typical examples of automatisms are the smacking of lips, fidgeting with clothing and wandering aimlessly.

Occasionally an automatism can result in a person being charged with a criminal offence such as shoplifting or even more serious offences. These charges are sometimes very difficult to defend and defendants need expert advice if they find themselves in such a position.

Benign Rolandic Epilepsy

This type of childhood epilepsy is most common in boys and usually strikes first between 2 and 10 years of age. The seizures are the most common type of simple partial seizures in childhood, affecting 15 -20% of children with epilepsy. Typically there will be a tingling sensation in the face or twitching of the face lips and tongue. These can cause speech arrest or slurring. During the seizure a certain amount of drooling might occur.

The prognosis is good.

Benzodiazepines

A class of drugs including - Mogadon®, Valium®, Rivotril® and Frisium®.

Blood Test

See Therapeutic Levels.

Brain The brain, situated inside the skull and made up of nerve cells called neurons, is the control centre for the nervous system.

The brain is divided into two sides known as the right and left hemispheres which are in turn divided into lobes.

The back of the brain, called the occipital lobe, controls vision.

The front of the brain is called the frontal lobe and this controls movement. The right frontal lobe controls movement on the left side of the body and the left frontal lobe controls movement on the right side of the body.

The middle part of the brain is called the temporal lobe and controls, for example, language, memory, emotions, heart rate and bowel function.

The brain is richly supplied by blood vessels. In fact, it consumes a quarter of the body's entire oxygen intake. This side view shows the left hemisphere, underneath which is the cerebellum, responsible for co-ordination of activities and balance.

The parietal lobe separates the frontal and occipital lobes and is responsible for processing sensory information and functions such as reading, as well as being the control centre for artistic and musical appreciation.

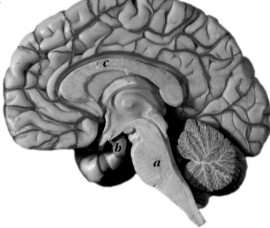

A cross section through the brain, showing the brain stem (a). The pituitary gland (b) lies underneath the centre of the brain. A thick bundle of nerves, the corpus callosum (c), joins the two hemispheres together. Compare this picture with the MRI scan on page 42.

At the base of the brain is the cerebellum which controls balance and regulates movement.

The maximum mass of brain tissue is reached at 20 years of age and then decreases steadily.

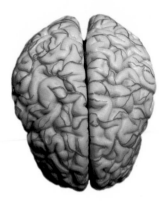

Break-through seizures These are seizures which occur unexpectedly following a long period of seizure control.

Top view of the brain showing the two hemispheres.

Breast Feeding Women with epilepsy can usually quite safely breast feed their babies. Fears that antiepileptic drugs are expressed in large quantities in breast milk and are transferred to affect the baby are largely unfounded. In fact, only minute traces of the most commonly used drugs are found in breast milk. The major exceptions to this general rule apply to phenobarbitone and ethosuximide which can be present in significant levels in breast milk. If the baby is subject to fairly high concentrations of phenobarbitone via breast milk it will become obviously drowsy and so bottle feeding is recommended.

For the mother who is anxious about dropping the baby during a seizure the best precaution is to sit on the floor with her back to the wall with cushions positioned on either side so that the baby will not have far to fall if the mother loses consciousness.

Carbamazepine The generic name of the antiepileptic drug Tegretol®.

Catalepsy A state where the muscles of the whole body remain in a semi rigid state which could last for several hours. It is not epilepsy.

Catamenial Seizures Seizures occurring around the time of the menstrual period. Another term used for these seizures is peri-menstrual seizures.

CAT Scan Computerized Axial Tomographic Scan. See CT scan.

Causes of Epilepsy There are two main causes of epilepsy:
- brain injury/disease and
- hereditary susceptibility

Brain injury or disease

- Damage to the brain with or without scarring as a result of:
    - (i) injury to the head
    - (ii) infections of the brain or brain meninges (encephalitis or meningitis)

- Malformation of the brain

- Degeneration of the brain

- Metabolic (biochemical) disorder as a result of:
    - (i) low blood glucose
    - (ii) low calcium level
    - (iii) drugs, particularly alcohol

- Brain tumours

Difficulties or problems during birth rarely cause epilepsy.

Hereditary Factors

See Genetic Inheritance

In generalised epilepsy hereditary factors are much more important than injury or disease.

In partial epilepsy injury or disease is more important than hereditary factors.

However, in many cases of both generalised and partial epilepsy neither set of factors seem important.

Cerebral lesion   A structural abnormality in the brain. The word "lesion" strictly means injury or damage but in modern terminology it is applied also to any area of abnormality.

Classification of Epilepsies   The International League Against Epilepsy (ILAE) recognised the need to clearly classify types of epilepsy to enable doctors across the world to discuss and study epilepsy in common terms. It therefore drew up a comprehensive table which took into account various syndromes which are determined by seizure types, age of onset, EEG abnormality and associated neurological features. The table is internationally recognised. It is important to doctors because it is used in predicting future progress, selecting the correct treatment and in helping to establish any underlying causes of seizures.

Classification of Seizures   The International League Against Epilepsy (ILAE) has determined a classification of seizures which divides seizure types into those which have a partial onset and those in which the onset is generalised. Partial seizures are further subdivided into simple partial seizures (where consciousness is retained throughout the seizure) and complex partial seizures (where at some time during seizures consciousness is impaired).

Partial Seizures

Simple Partial
(consciousness not impaired)

a) with motor symptoms
b) with sensory symptoms
c) with autonomic symptoms
d) with psychic symptoms
It is possible for simple partial seizures to develop into complex partial seizures.

Complex Partial Seizures
(consciousness is impaired)

a) with impairment of consciousness only
b) with automatisms

It is possible for partial seizures, especially complex partial, to develop into tonic-clonic generalised seizures. Such seizures are known as **Secondarily Generalised Seizures.**

Generalised Seizures

(consciousness is always impaired)

Typical Absence seizures

Atypical Absence seizures

Myoclonic seizures

Clonic seizures

Tonic seizures

Tonic Clonic seizures

Atonic seizures

Clobazam The generic name of an antiepileptic drug Frisium®.

Clonazepam The generic name of an antiepileptic drug Rivotril®.

Clonic movements These are twitches and generalised rhythmic movements of the muscles.

Clonic Seizures These are generalised seizures in which the muscles contract and relax continuously causing the person having the seizure to twitch and jerk repeatedly.

Complex Absence Seizures These seizures have been renamed, now being known as atypical absence seizures, and occur across the whole age range with people who have some form of brain damage. The seizures last longer than simple absence seizures and result in massive jerks or a very sudden loss of muscle tone - either of which can cause the person to fall to the ground with some force. They injure may themselves in the process and many have to wear protective headgear to avoid head injuries.

Complex Partial Seizures These types of partial seizure usually originate in the temporal lobes of the brain and are non convulsive in nature. They differ from simple partial seizures because they produce impaired or altered consciousness. Epilepsy with these types of seizure is also know as Temporal Lobe Epilepsy (TLE) or Psychomotor Epilepsy.

As the temporal lobes are such complex parts of the brain, controlling such things as the sense of smell, the sense of taste, visual and musical appreciation and the "inbuilt time clock" it is no surprise that when something goes awry in this part of the brain the results can be chaotic.

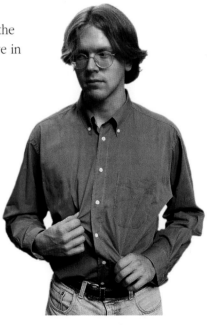

These seizures often commence with a simple partial seizure (called an aura) in which the person becomes disorientated. He/she may pluck at clothing or smack lips and perhaps wander aimlessly about the room.

Random plucking at clothing can be a typical feature of a complex partial seizure.

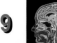

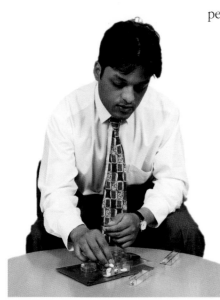

People who have this type of seizure tend to be quite relieved when they are told what is happening to them. They are relieved because the problem is purely physical in nature and nothing to do with their mental state.

It is essential that the physician treating the person is aware of all the symptoms so that a correct diagnosis can be made and the most effective medication be prescribed.

Compliance In a medical context the word applies to the ability and willingness to take prescribed medication. One of the most common causes of "break through" seizures is the failure to take antiepileptic drugs. This inevitably leads to an increased seizure pattern or a return of seizures when the person has enjoyed a long period of being seizure free.

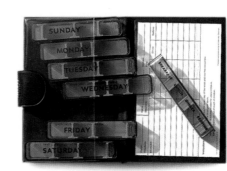

Compliance can be improved by using a specially designed tablet container (sometimes known as a "dosette"). It is easy to see at a glance whether the correct dose has been taken at the correct time.

Contraception and epilepsy The effectiveness of the oral contraceptive pill can be adversely affected by some antiepileptic drugs. This is because many antiepileptic drugs cause other drugs taken at the same time to be destroyed too rapidly in the liver. This can cause contraception to fail.

Sexually active women, who have epilepsy and are taking antiepileptic drugs alongside the oral contraceptive pill as the only means of contraception, should consult their doctors. In virtually all cases the risk of an unwanted pregnancy can be overcome by making adjustments to the type of contraceptive pill taken.

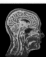

Convulsion This is the term used to describe what is commonly perceived as an epileptic attack in which the limbs become rigid and shake. A convulsion can last for anything up to 5 minutes without causing undue concern. If, however, the convulsion lasts longer than 5 minutes a serious medical condition called "status epilepticus" could develop and medical help should be sought.

Many people with epilepsy do have convulsions. They can also occur in very young babies when there is a rapid and sustained rise in body temperature. These are called febrile convulsions and because they are usually isolated episodes they are not classified as being epileptic seizures.

CT Scan Computerised Tomographic Scan (also known as a CAT scan). It is an X-ray test which provides detailed pictures of cross sections of the brain. It is important to be aware that only a relatively small proportion of people 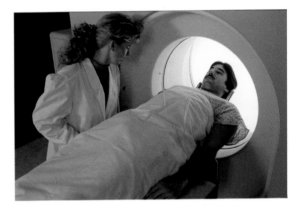 with epilepsy require a CT Scan (also known as a CAT Scan) as part of the routine investigations.

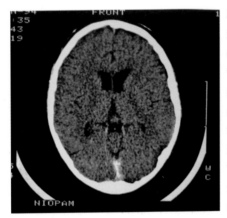

Scans take place at a hospital radiology department and are carried out by a radiographer who will report to a consultant radiologist. A scan involves lying down on a bed which moves towards the scanner so that the head is surrounded by the machinery. The person lies still for some minutes whilst a series of x-rays are taken. The procedure is brief and

A typical CAT scan showing a cross section through the head, as seen from above.

 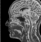

involves no physical discomfort, though some people do feel somewhat uncomfortable at being enclosed within the scanner. Also an injection is sometimes necessary to provide a contrast on the scanned image.

The images taken during the scan are enhanced through a computer and transferred to conventional X-ray film to be read by a neuro-radiologist. The images and the neuro-radiologist's report are then passed to the consultant physician who requested the scan.

Déja vu This is a common expression used to describe a feeling that one is repeating a previous experience, for example when visiting a place for the first time. This can be quite disconcerting, but is relevant in the diagnosis and treatment of epilepsy because such feelings often signal the start of a complex partial seizure. Such an episode is called an "aura". Most people experience déja vu at some time or other but with people who have complex partial seizures it can be very prominent and a feature of their epilepsy.

Diazemuls® A trade name of the antiepileptic drug diazepam.

Diazepam The generic name of drugs Valium®, Diazemuls® or Stesolid®.

These drugs do not prevent the onset of seizures but are successful when used to stop prolonged seizures which are in progress ("status epilepticus"). They can be given intravenously or, more commonly, rectally, using a special applicator to introduce the drug directly.

Differential Diagnosis It is quite common for other disorders to be mistaken for epilepsy, because they exhibit some of the same symptoms. Typical examples range from simple faints, panic attacks and vertigo through to pseudoseizures. As a result, the diagnosis of epilepsy is incorrectly made and antiepileptic drugs are prescribed which are not at all necessary. To ensure that the correct diagnosis is given it is advisable to have a diagnosis confirmed by a consultant neurologist or a physician with a special interest in epilepsy.

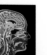

Diurnal Seizures   These are seizures which occur during waking hours, in contrast to nocturnal seizures which occur during sleeping hours.

Domestic Hazards   Because the onset of seizures is generally unpredictable there are certain hazards from seizures which need to be guarded against. One of the most delicate situations concerns bathing and privacy. It is a sad fact that people have died in the bath during a seizure and, therefore, some sensible safety precautions have to be taken. These are straightforward and should preserve privacy:

- tell responsible people in the household of the intention to take a bath
- make sure that the water is not too deep
- make sure that the water is not so hot as to induce sleep
- leave the bathroom door unlocked so that discreet supervision is at hand.

If someone does have a seizure in the bath:

- remove the plug and clear the plug hole of obstructions
- hold the head above water
- call for assistance if this is required and available
- try to prevent injury (use bath towels etc.)
- keep the person warm
- do not attempt to lift the person out of the bath until fully recovered
- take care not to slip on the wet floor.

An alternative to bathing is to have a shower. The danger of drowning is removed, although injury is still possible within the shower cubicle.

The following precautions should reduce any risk:

- if possible inform other people of the intention to take a shower
- leave the shower room door unlocked
- take a small seat into the shower and sit under the fall of water.

Poorly maintained gas appliances are a danger to all people but especially to people with epilepsy. It is absolutely essential to ensure that all automatic ignition systems are in perfect working order.

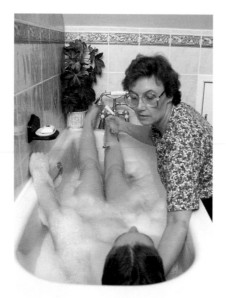

Drain the water out of the bath.

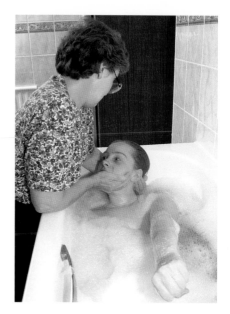

Keep supporting the head until the seizure stops.

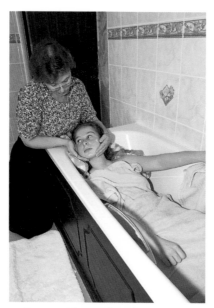

Cover with towels to keep warm.

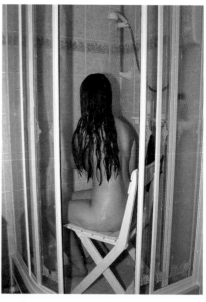

In showers, use a chair to reduce the dangers of falling during a seizure.

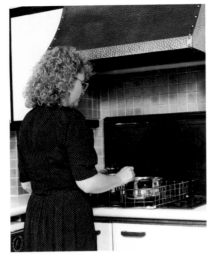

A cooker guard dramatically reduces the risk of serious injury.

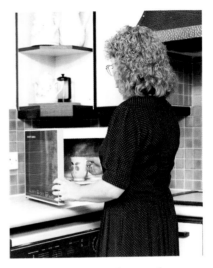

Microwave cooking, where possible, is even safer.

It is also possible to suffocate on a pillow if a seizure occurs whilst asleep and an anti-suffocation pillow is to be strongly recommended. Names and addresses of suppliers of these pillows can be obtained from the Epilepsy Associations.

The dangers of a seizure near to a cooking appliance are obvious and so special precautions should be taken. A specially constructed cooker guard - a bit awkward to work with but infinitely better than risking serious injury - can be obtained from all major stores dealing in cooking appliances or child-care products.

It is essential that gas appliances are regularly maintained by a qualified gas engineer.

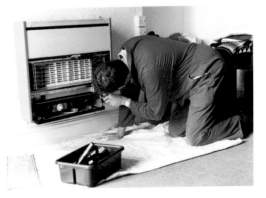

Driving

The regulations in the UK governing the issue of driving licences to people with a history of epilepsy are quite specific. They are split into two categories, viz an Ordinary Driving Entitlement and a Vocational Driving Entitlement.

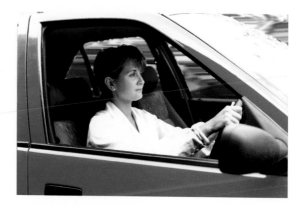

For an ordinary entitlement the person who has epilepsy may qualify for a driving licence if he or she has been free from any epileptic attack for one year. (An epileptic attack is interpreted as any seizure involving episodes such as limbs jerking, auras or absences and need not necessarily involve a loss of consciousness.)

A person who cannot meet these conditions may qualify for an ordinary driving licence provided that he or she has established over a period of at least three years (beginning on the date of an asleep attack), a history or pattern of attacks which occur only when asleep.

In either case, the applicant or licence holder suffering from epilepsy must not be regarded as a likely source of danger to the public as a driver.

If while holding a driving licence a driver suffers from an epileptic attack, driving must cease immediately (unless the sleep regulations can be met) and Driver and Vehicle Licensing Agency (DVLA) be notified.

For a Vocational Entitlement demanding either a Large Goods Vehicle (LGV) licence or a Passenger Carrying Vehicle (PCV) licence, drivers must satisfy all the following conditions:

- hold a full ordinary driving licence
- have been free of an epileptic attack for at least the last ten years
- have not taken antiepileptic drugs during this ten year period
- do not have a continuing liability to epileptic seizure.

The duty of informing the licensing authority of an onset of seizures clearly lies with the applicant or the licence holder because it is that person who knowingly puts others at risk.

Doctors have a duty to inform patients that they should not drive when in the doctor's opinion it would be dangerous to do so. The British Medical Association in its ethical guidelines clearly advises doctors to actively encourage patients to inform the licensing authorities and to indicate that they will do so themselves if the patient continues to drive. Furthermore, they should ask patients to return after considering the matter and inform them of the action they have taken. In exceptional circumstances doctors may consider breaching confidentiality in the public interest if they deem this appropriate.

The withdrawal of a licence is not automatic since provision is made for the person to seek a second medical opinion and an independent assessment of driving competence.

The regulations in the Republic of Ireland vary from those operating in the UK. The conditions for which a person with epilepsy can drive are laid out in the Road Traffic Act (Licensing of Drivers) Regulations 1989 viz.:

- a person who has been free of epileptic attacks for two years can be granted a licence to drive a car, light van, tractor or motorcycle
- a person who has epilepsy or who has a history of epilepsy will not be granted a licence to drive larger vehicles such as lorries and buses.

In other countries other regulations may exist. It is important to be informed before going abroad by car.

The International Bureau for Epilepsy (IBE) has published a report by the ILAE/IBE Commission on Driving Licensing named "Epilepsy and Driving Licence Regulations".

Drop Attacks These generalised seizures are otherwise known as atonic seizures.

Drug Interactions It is possible for some drugs to adversely affect other drugs. One example of this is the neutralising effect of some antiepileptic drugs on the oral contraceptive pill causing contraception to fail.

Drug Side Effects All drugs have side effects and those developed for control of seizures are no exception. Because some side effects of antiepileptic drugs can be alarming and unpleasant it is essential that patients should be familiar with them. Ideally, doctors should advise as to the nature of likely adverse reactions. If doctors do not volunteer the information the patient should ask. Local pharmacists are also usually very helpful.

Women of child-bearing age who have epilepsy should be aware that some antiepileptic drugs can harm a developing foetus. They should seek advice if they are contemplating pregnancy or are pregnant.

By 1999 legislation will be fully in place to ensure that patient information leaflets are issued with all prescribed medicines and these will give information about side effects.

Education

The vast majority of children who have epilepsy attend mainstream schools being accepted as normal children who happen to have epilepsy. They invariably follow the full National Curriculum. Some areas of the curriculum can present problems such as certain aspects of physical education, one of which is swimming. However, these problems are usually and effectively overcome. Very often a provision of attendance at a mainstream school is that the teaching and non-teaching staff have a working knowledge of first aid procedures in the event of a pupil having a seizure.

Many young people with epilepsy progress through statutory schooling with few problems and do well in public examinations. Examination Boards do have special provision for those whose results are adversely affected by a medical condition.

There is a higher prevalence of epilepsy amongst children attending schools catering for pupils with learning and or behavioural difficulties. This is to be expected - the cause of the learning or behavioural difficulties is also quite likely to have some bearing on the cause of the epilepsy.

Disability, including epilepsy, need be no barrier to further or higher education. Students with epilepsy should target courses which they know they are capable of undertaking from both a physical and academic point of view.

For the small proportion of children who have severe intractable epilepsy special provision is made in residential schools which cater especially for their needs. At present there are three schools in the United Kingdom which fill this specialised role. They are:

St. Pier's School
Lingfield
Surrey RH7 6PW
Tel: 01342 832243

St. Elizabeth's School
Much Hadham
Herts SG10 6EW
Tel: 0127984 3451

The David Lewis School
David Lewis Centre
Warford
Cheshire SK9 7UD
Tel: 01565 872613

EEG (Electroencephalogram)

The brain emits minute amounts of electricity throughout the day and the electroencephalogram is a machine that amplifies this electricity to produce a graphical trace called an electroencephalograph (EEG).

Electrodes are fixed to the scalp using an adhesive and recordings are made of the brain's electrical activity to determine the type of trace made from specific parts of the brain. A neurologist or a neurophysiologist will study the traces made to establish if any abnormality is present.

The test does not cause any discomfort since it is merely recording the electrical activity of the brain and no electricity passes from the machine to the brain.

On very rare occasions and for specific reasons the electrodes may be placed on the brain surface using a surgical procedure. If this technique is used, the person being tested is anaesthetised and so is unaware of what is happening.

The EEG machine is used to assist neurologists in determining the type of epilepsy an individual may have. A common misconception is that recordings can confirm or deny the existence of epilepsy. This is not the case and the most important thing which helps the neurologist get the right diagnosis is a good eye-witness account of the episodes.

E

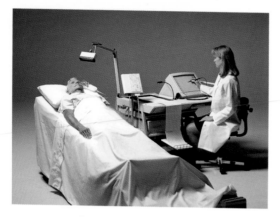

A modern EEG machine with both conventional paper traces and digital on-screen facilities.

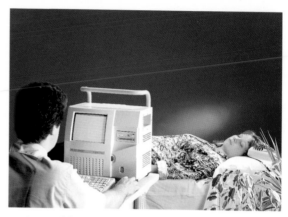

A portable EEG machine which can be used in areas where EEG tests are not normally carried out.

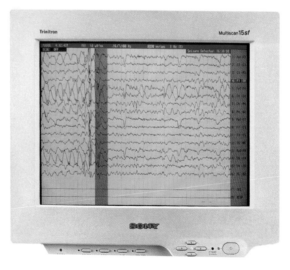

Close up of on-screen EEG trace.

EEG (Electroencephalograph)

This is the tracing of the brainwaves recorded by the electroencephalogram.

Until recently the graphs were always drawn on to paper but some specialised units now use electroencephalograms which are paper-free and the traces are viewed on a visual display unit.

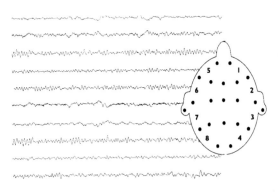

A normal EEG trace.

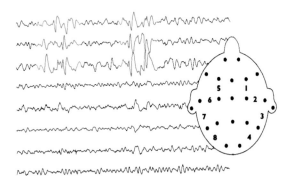

The red areas show electrical disturbances in someone with simple partial seizures.

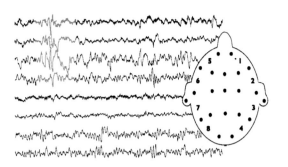

The red areas show electrical disturbances in someone who has complex partial seizures.

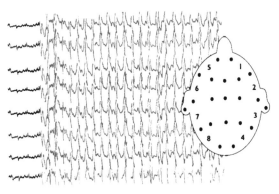

The red areas show electrical disturbances over the whole brain, indicating a typical absence seizure.

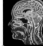

Emeside® The trade name for the antiepileptic drug ethosuximide.

Employment Most jobs, covering the total range of ability and disability should be available for people with epilepsy. Examples of suitable work are:

- the professions, including: Medicine, Accountancy and the Law
- public service, including: teaching*, civil service and local government (*Applicants for teacher training should have been free from seizures for 2 years at the time of applying)
- general office work
- general labouring
- a vast amount of occupations in service industries.

There are, however, occupations which are unsuitable for people with epilepsy. Examples are:

- Aircraft Pilot (applicants shall have no established medical history or clinical diagnosis of epilepsy)
- Armed Services
  Army (applicants are rejected on the grounds of epilepsy)
  Navy (medical regulations state that any seizures at any age debar entry)
  Air Force (proven epilepsy with few exceptions is a bar to recruitment)
- Deep Sea Diving (a history of seizures, apart from febrile convulsions, will preclude granting of a Certificate of Fitness to Dive)
- Emergency Services
  Police (applicants currently having seizures are not recruited - those with a past history are dealt with on an individual basis)

  Fire (a history of epilepsy renders a person unsuitable for operational fire duties - those who have been free of seizures from childhood may be considered individually)

  Ambulance (in order to qualify as a driver applicants should be free from any epileptic seizure and off antiepileptic medication for 10 years or more and they must pass a medical examination)

- Merchant Navy (absolute barrier for applicants with a history of seizures since the age of 5 years)

- Prison Officer (recent history of seizures debars an applicant on the grounds of security from posts at Prison Officer Grades, but applicants to other grades of prison service are considered individually)

- Train Driver (absolute barrier if seizures have occurred after the age of 5 years).

It is sometimes advisable to be registered as disabled. The statutory employment services can provide guidance as to the advantages and disadvantages of registration.

Epanutin® The trade name for the antiepileptic drug phenytoin.

Epilepsy The name given to a nervous disorder which affects about 1 person in every 150 of the population, making it the most common of all neurological disorders.

The condition can affect anyone at any time. Many famous people throughout the ages have been known to have epilepsy, amongst them wonderful musicians, great leaders and those who excel at sport.

Epilepsy manifests itself in many different ways, ranging from dramatic convulsive episodes to simple apparently innocuous blank stares as well as many other manifestations.

These epileptic episodes are called seizures and are symptomatic of some form of brain disorder. They arise when there is an abnormal disorganised burst of electrical activity either across the whole brain or in a localised area of the brain.

An internationally accepted Classification of Seizures defines seizure types into two main divisions, generalised seizures and partial seizures. The partial seizures are further subdivided into simple partial seizures and complex partial seizures.

A diagnosis of epilepsy is usually only made following a series of seizures.

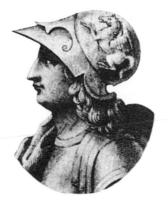

Alexander the Great

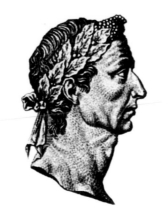

Julius Caesar

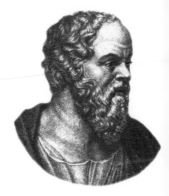

Socrates

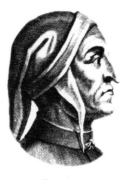

Dante

There is clear evidence
that many great historical
figures had epilepsy. Just
a few are shown here.

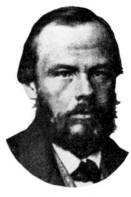

Dostoevsky

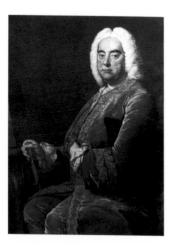

Handel

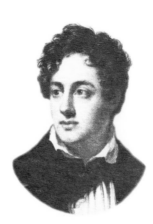

Byron

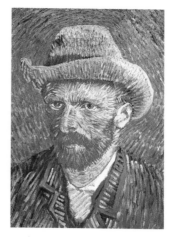

Van Gogh

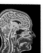

The aim of treatment is to completely control the seizures and is, in the vast majority of cases, carried out using antiepileptic drugs.

The condition can, in certain cases, also be treated by surgery. This method of treatment is only used when the seizures cannot be controlled by drugs and the person's epilepsy renders itself suitable for surgical intervention.

Although it is not always possible, a diagnosis of epilepsy should always be confirmed either by a consultant neurologist or a doctor who has a special interest in epilepsy, to ensure that the correct diagnosis is made.

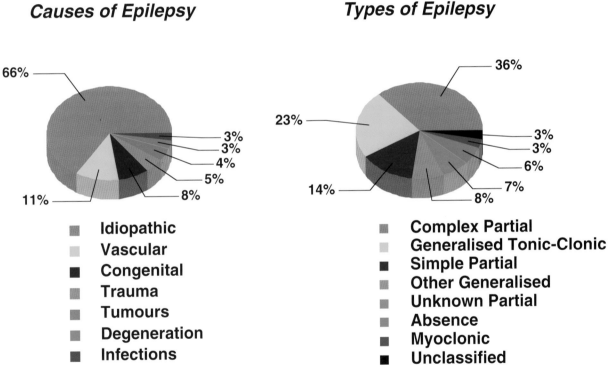

Causes of Epilepsy

66%
3%
3%
4%
5%
11%
8%

■ Idiopathic
■ Vascular
■ Congenital
■ Trauma
■ Tumours
■ Degeneration
■ Infections

Types of Epilepsy

36%
23%
3%
3%
6%
14%
7%
8%

■ Complex Partial
■ Generalised Tonic-Clonic
■ Simple Partial
■ Other Generalised
■ Unknown Partial
■ Absence
■ Myoclonic
■ Unclassified

Epilepsy Associations

These are voluntary bodies which exist to improve the quality of life of people with epilepsy.

They are organised into two main sectors. One works to support people with epilepsy in the community and the other specifically cares for people with epilepsy in a residential setting. Both sectors come together regularly under the umbrella of the Joint Epilepsy Council of the UK and Ireland (JEC).

There are six member Associations of the JEC which work tirelessly to promote positive attitudes towards epilepsy by such activities as providing support groups, social worker support and counselling services, education programmes, funding for research projects and a vast amount of educational literature.

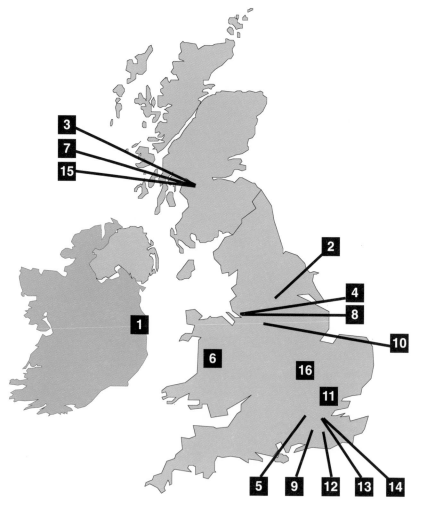

1. Brainwave
The Irish Epilepsy Association
249 Crumlin Road
Dublin
Tel: Dublin 4557500
Fax: Dublin 4557013

2. British Epilepsy Association
Anstey House
40 Hanover Square
Leeds LS3 1BE
Tel: 0113 2439393
Fax: 0113 2428804
Helpline: 0800 30 90 30
E-mail: epilepsy@bea.org.uk

3. Epilepsy Association of Scotland
48 Govan Road
Glasgow G51 1JL
Tel: 0141 427 4911
Fax: 0141 427 7414

4. Mersey Region Epilepsy Association
The Glaxo Neurological Centre
Norton Street
Liverpool L3 8LR
Tel: 0151 298 2666
Fax: 0151 298 2333

5. The National Society for Epilepsy
Chalfont Centre for Epilepsy
Chalfont St. Peter
Gerards Cross
Buckinghamshire SL9 0RJ
Tel: (General) 01494 601300
        (Helpline) 01494 601400

6. Epilepsi Cymru: Epilepsy Wales
Gwynedd Voluntary Services Council
Eldon Square
Dolgellau
Gwynedd Tel: 01341 422575

In addition there are a number of organisations which would be delighted to offer guidance and advice on available services and facilities:

7. Quarriers Village Epilepsy Centre
Bridge of Weir
Renfewshire PA11 3SA
Tel: 01505 612224

8. The Maghull Homes
Liverpool Road South
Maghull
Liverpool L31 8BR
Tel: 0151 526 4133
Fax: 0151 526 1118

9. Meath Home
Westbrook Road
Godalming
Surrey GU7 2QJ
Tel: 01483 415095
Fax: 01483 414101

10. The David Lewis Centre
Alderley Edge
Cheshire
Tel: 01565 872613

11. St. Elizabeth's Home and School
Much Hadham
Herts. SG10 6EW
Tel: 0127984 3451

12. St. Piers Lingfield
St. Piers Lane
Lingfield
Surrey RH7 6PW
Tel: 01342 832243
Fax 01342 834639

All of the organisations listed above are members of the JEC (Joint Epilepsy Council of the UK and Ireland). Other members of the JEC are:

13. Centre for Epilepsy
Maudsley Hospital
Denmark Hill
London SE5 8AZ Tel: 0171
703 6333

14. The Epilepsy Research Foundation (ERF)
PO Box 3004
London W4 1XT
Tel/Fax 0181 995 4781

15. Epilepsy Research Group
University Department of Medicine and Therapeutics
Gardner Institute
Western Infirmary
Glasgow G11 6NT Tel: 0141 211 2572

16. Epilepsy Specialist Nurses Association
Department of Neurology
Northampton General Hospital
NN1 5BD
Tel: 01604 34700 (extension 4926)

Some of the organisations listed above are actively involved in the work of the International Bureau for Epilepsy (IBE).

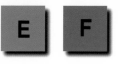

Epilepsy Specialist Nurse These are nurses who have had specialist training in dealing with problems associated with epilepsy. They work alongside doctors and other health professionals, usually in hospital specialist epilepsy units. Very often they sit in with the consultant neurologists at outpatient clinics and their work extends beyond the clinic into the home and work places.

Epilim® The trade name of the antiepileptic drug sodium valproate.

Epilim Chrono® The trade name of a slow release preparation of the antiepileptic drug sodium valproate.

Ethosuximide This is the generic name for the antiepileptic drugs Emeside® and Zarontin®.

Febrile Convulsions These occur most commonly between the ages of six months and five years. They occur only when a child has a raised temperature higher than 38^0 C (the normal body temperature being 37^0 C). Sometimes a convulsion is the first indication that a child is developing a febrile illness.

Approximately 3% of all children experience febrile convulsions. In about a third of these cases, there is a near relative with a similar history.

Only 5% of children who have febrile convulsions are likely to develop epilepsy in later life.

First Aid The following practical steps to be taken in the event of a seizure are simple and straightforward. When the seizure starts:

- keep calm
- clear a space around the person, moving objects that may be harmful
- reassure others and explain what you are doing
- make the person comfortable by lying him/her down, easing from a chair only if necessary
- cushion the head to prevent facial injury
- loosen tight neckwear - remove spectacles and high heeled shoes, if worn.

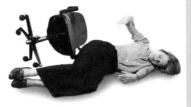

Seizures can appear alarming. It is essential for onlookers to remain calm.

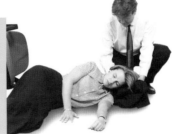

If possible, support the head with something soft to prevent injury.

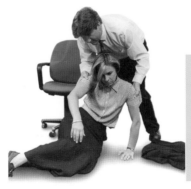

When the seizure is over help the person to a position where recovery can take place.

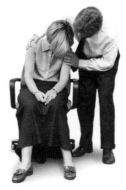

Reassure the person as recovery continues.

When the movements have stopped:

- turn the person on the side (first aid recovery position)
- wipe away any excess saliva from the mouth, check that dentures or vomit are not blocking the throat.

Some people have seizures which put them temporarily out of touch with their surroundings. Behaviour may appear strange to the observer - for example, the person may wander around aimlessly with glazed expression. During this type of seizure the person should be accompanied and gently led away from any source of danger.

At the end of the seizure:

- reassure the person if there is confusion and explain what has happened
- check for obvious injury
- observe and stay with the person until recovery is complete.

Assistance may be needed to secure a safe return to routine or to a place of safety. Provide privacy and offer assistance if there has been incontinence.

DO NOT put anything in the mouth.

DO NOT restrain or restrict movements during the seizure.

DO NOT give anything to drink.

DO NOT move unless in danger.

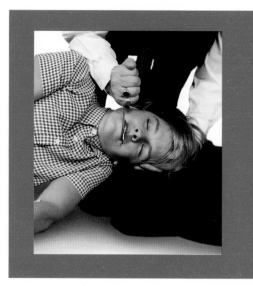

Never place anything into the mouth at any stage of a seizure. A bitten tongue will heal - broken teeth will not.

Fits   The word often used in place of "seizures".

Focal Motor Seizures   These are simple partial seizures which cause movement of the limbs, head or neck and they originate in the frontal lobes of the brain. If the seizure is in the right frontal lobe then seizure movement is produced on the left side of the body and vice versa. This usually results in what is called an adversive seizure.

A rare type of focal motor seizure begins with a simple twitch of the thumb of one hand. The twitching develops into a jerking and spreads to the whole hand, the whole arm, the face and finally to the leg. This type of seizure is sometimes called a "Jacksonian Seizure" because it was the British neurologist John Hughlings Jackson (1835 -1911) who first described it. When the jerking has spread to the whole side of the body it is possible for the person to lose consciousness and progress to a typical tonic-clonic seizure. This tonic-clonic seizure is said to be a secondarily generalised seizure.

Seizures originating in the frontal lobe can also involve an interruption in speech.

Focal Sensory Seizures   These simple partial seizures originate in the parietal lobes of the brain, producing physical sensations such as tingling or an unnatural warmth. If the seizure is in the right parietal lobe it will manifest itself as a tingling or warmth on the left hand side of the body and vice versa. Seizures originating in the frontal lobe can also involve an interruption in speech.

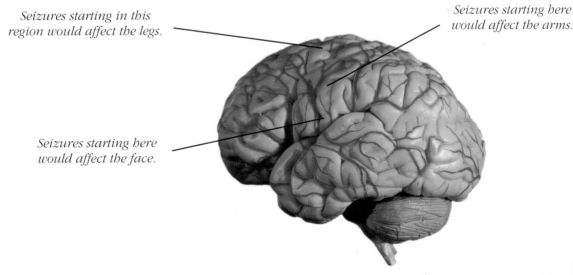

Seizures starting in this region would affect the legs.

Seizures starting here would affect the arms.

Seizures starting here would affect the face.

Folic Acid See Pregnancy and Epilepsy

Frisium® The trade name for the antiepileptic drug clobazam

Frontal Lobe Seizures Seizures originating from the frontal lobes of the brain. See Focal Motor Seizures and Complex Partial Seizures

Gabapentin The generic name of the antiepileptic drug Neurontin®

Gabatril® The trade name of the drug tiagabine which is currently being developed and tested prior to being licensed.

Gamma-amino butyric acid GABA is a naturally occurring chemical in the brain and has the effect of reducing in the brain the levels of excitability of nerve cells. Some modern antiepileptic drugs are designed to increase the activity of GABA so as to prevent seizures.

Generalised Seizures With this type of seizure the whole brain is affected by abnormal electrical disturbance and the person becomes unconscious of surroundings. Examples of generalised seizures are: tonic clonic seizures, absence seizures, myoclonic/jerk seizures.

When the onset of such seizures is immediate the seizures are said to be generalised and when they progress from partial seizures they are said to be secondarily generalised.

Generic Name of Drug This is the chemical name of a drug as opposed to its trade name. Generally speaking, the medical profession invariably refer to a drug by its generic name (e.g. vigabatrin) whereas the public refers to its trade name (Sabril®).

Genetic Inheritance Epilepsy can be genetically inherited but more commonly there is no family history of epilepsy. Some types of generalised epilepsies such as absence epilepsy, juvenile myoclonic epilepsy and generalised tonic-clonic seizures on awakening, are hereditary. In the majority of cases, however, inheritance probably plays only a limited role and this is especially true of partial seizures. It is assumed that contributions made by the father and the mother in relation to the inheritance of epilepsy are of equal importance.

Grand Mal Seizures

See tonic-clonic seizures

Heredity Factors

See Genetic Inheritance

History of Epilepsy

The "Sacred Disease" or epilepsy as it called today is as old as the human race. As early as 2080 BC, Hammurabi, King of Babylon, made mention of it in his laws. Then, as now, it assumed both medical and social importance. The laws demonstrated that prejudice existed even then against the person with epilepsy.

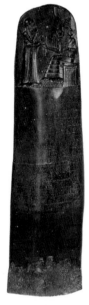

The code of Hammurabi. The stone pillar is on display in the Louvre.

For example, two sections of the Code of Hammurabi meant that a person with epilepsy was not allowed to marry and could not act as a member of a jury or as a witness in a court of law.

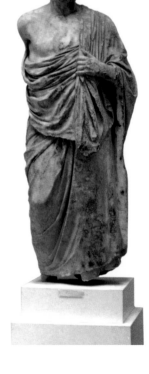

Hippocrates - the Father of Medicine

The Hippocratic collection of medical writings - "On the Sacred Disease" (circa 400 BC), did at least attempt a scientific explanation for epilepsy, in contrast to previous superstitions. The explanation was that epilepsy is caused by an excess of phlegm. Superstition remained, however, and many strange customs evolved. A Roman custom was to spit on seeing an epileptic seizure in the belief that this would keep the demon away and thus avoid infection. The Romans called this condition 'morbis comitialis', meaning that it interrupted the proceedings of the 'comitia', i.e. the assembly of the people. An explanation of the name given comes from the writings of the poet physician of the 3rd century, Quintus Serenus:

"A kind of sudden sickness, 'tis, whose name has clung since the votes of a true count it prevents ..."

For people with epilepsy life was miserable and they were subject to extreme degradation. To the public they were merely objects of horror and disgust. The Roman author, Apuleius, when writing about a slave boy, Thallus, said that fellow slaves would have nothing to do with him because of his epilepsy.

"Nobody dares to eat with him from the same dish or drink from the same cup lest he contaminate the family"

Epilepsy also occurs in the Bible. The following passage from the New Testament (Mark 14-29) gives an accurate description of a tonic-clonic seizure and clearly illustrates the popular view that epileptic children were suffering from demoniacal possession.

"When they rejoined the disciples they saw a large crowd around them and some scribes arguing with them. When they saw him the whole crowd were struck with amazement and ran to greet him. 'What are you arguing about with them?" he asked.

A man answered from the crowd: "Master, I have brought my son to you; there is a spirit of dumbness in him, and when it takes hold of him it throws him to the ground, and he foams at the mouth and grinds his teeth and goes rigid. And I asked your disciples to cast it out and they were unable to." "You faithless generation" he said to them in reply. "How much longer must I be with you? How much longer must I put up with you? Bring him to me." They brought the boy to him and as soon as the spirit saw Jesus it threw the boy into convulsions, and he fell on the ground and lay writhing there, foaming at the mouth. Jesus asked the father, "How long has this been happening to him?" "From childhood," he replied, "and often it has thrown him into fire and into water, in order to destroy him. But if you can do anything, have pity and help us." And when Jesus saw how many people were pressing round him he rebuked the unclean spirit. "Deaf and dumb spirit", he said, "I command you : come out of him and never enter him again." Then throwing the boy into violent convulsions it came out shouting and the boy lay there so like a corpse that many of them said "He

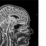

is dead." But Jesus took him by the hand and helped him up, and he was able to stand."

A misconception that epilepsy was a form of lunacy existed in the 2nd and 3rd centuries. Both philosophers and physicians connected the condition with lunar phases, as indeed they did with many other illnesses.

With the spread of Christianity, saints were adopted as being patrons of those afflicted with what was by now called the "falling sickness". The most popular of these saints was Saint Valentine. Pilgrims were taken to the Priory of St. Valentine in the hope of finding a cure. Many devotional rites were followed, the centre of these being a celebration of as many as three masses. Hospitals for people with epilepsy were built at such places of pilgrimage.

Treatment of the condition became wide and varied. One of the most bizarre set of instructions for dealing with a person during a seizure was written by a fifteenth century lecturer in medicine, Antonius Guainerius:

" If a paroxism comes to an epileptic, let it be your aim to prevent the ascent of vapours, and so far as possible to draw the matter downwards. Therefore perform painful ligatures on the extremities, on the buttocks, under the knee make a slight incision with a cupping glass; and call the patient in a loud voice by his own name - place a wooden peg between his teeth - also at once kill a dog, and give the gall to the patient in any way that you can. If the first one who sees the attack urinates in his own shoe and then stirs it around as if to wash it, then afterwards the patient will be entirely delivered."

He also made recommendations for treatment to be taken during seizure free periods. Here the unfortunate person was instructed to...

"avoid fear, sadness, anger and all disturbances of soul; also coitus, unless he be a robust youth accustomed to it; he may then have intercourse lest his semen be turned into poison by being too long retained."

It was recommended that tablets could solve all other problems of any curable epilepsy. These tablets were to be made from substances such as "... the rib of the left side of a man who has been hanged or beheaded and give it to the patient every morning for a month; it should be taken with water."

It is probably fair to say that none of these remedies was particularly successful.

Surgical methods of curing epilepsy were primitive in medieval times. The most popular course of action was cauterisation in which hot irons were applied to the head and surrounding areas. Perhaps more logically, the practice arose of making a hole in the head so that offending matter could make its escape.

By the seventeenth century, physicians would no longer use methods such as those described by Guainerius. While the search went on for a greater understanding and a more successful form of therapy, physicians stopped using such materials as blood, urine and dung etc.

General attitudes towards the epileptic patient gradually improved during the 18th century. The popular belief that epilepsy was infectious (which is even held in some parts of the world today!) was being scientifically disproven and patients were no longer locked in wards in appalling conditions. The sight of the epileptic patient being shackled to the wall became mercifully more infrequent.

It was in the 19th century that the first major breakthrough in antiepileptic therapy was achieved. The discovery of potassium bromide as an antiepileptic drug occurred by accident. It was popularly supposed by Victorian moralists that epilepsy was a result of excess sexual activity and for males with epilepsy castration was the only true cure.

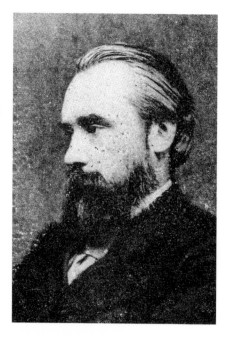

John Hughlings Jackson (1835 - 1911)

In the National Hospital, Queen's Square, London, patients suffering from sexually transmitted diseases were being treated with bromide which causes temporary impotence. It was noted that patients who also had epilepsy showed a marked decrease in seizure pattern. Hence the discovery of the first truly antiepileptic drug. It became so popular that enormous doses of bromide were being prescribed - at one stage 2 tons of bromide were

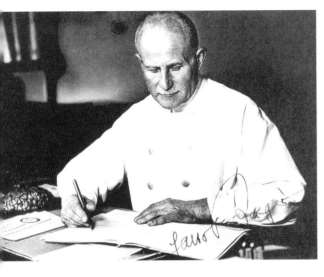

Hans Berger (1873 - 1941), inventor of the electroencephalogram.

being used annually in the treatment of epilepsy at the National Hospital alone. Unfortunately, there were drug side effects which are best described by quoting from Hammond, as he exhibited a patient in New York:

"As you see he is broken down in appearance, has large abscesses in his neck and is altogether in a bad condition. But this is better than to have epilepsy."

Most people did not agree that these side effects were better than having epilepsy and so the use of the drug was gradually withdrawn.

At about the same time a German scientist, Van Boyer, was experimenting with the drug phenobarbitone. He was using this drug as a sedative and in this sphere it was very successful. It was not until 1912, however, that another German, Alfred Hauptman, advocated its use as an antiepileptic drug. It proved to be a great success in early effective treatment.

Probably one of the greatest contributions to a better understanding of epilepsy was made by an English neurologist, John Hughlings Jackson who published the findings of his work in 1870. His interest in the condition was stimulated by a form of epilepsy demonstrated by his wife. Her seizures were focal motor seizures and today the condition is sometimes referred to as Jacksonian Epilepsy.

In 1929 Hans Berger discovered that the minute electrical discharges from the brain could be recorded and measured on a machine called an electroencephalogram. This represented a huge advance in diagnostic technique.

In 1950 the British Epilepsy Association was formed to promote a better understanding of the condition and since then advances in every sphere have been rapid. New hi-tech diagnostic equipment such as CAT Scanners and MRI Scanners have enabled doctors to pinpoint areas of the brain from which seizures may originate. Surgery has advanced beyond all recognition and new drugs have been developed to give a greater degree of control.

Despite all the advances in medical knowledge and improvement in a public understanding of epilepsy there is still much work to be done.

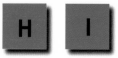
Hyperventilation This simply means over-breathing and can be a significant factor in provoking absence seizures in children. Only very rarely does hyperventilation provoke a tonic-clonic seizure.

During a routine EEG test a patient will be asked to blow deeply and rapidly to see if it results in any significant change in the trace being recorded and give a possible indication of triggering a seizure.

IBE International Bureau for Epilepsy - an organisation founded to improve the quality of life of people with epilepsy through a better understanding of epilepsy and to improve the social consequences of epilepsy throughout the world. It produces a lot of educational material and organises many conferences and educational events. The Headquarters of the IBE is in the Netherlands, located at PO Box 21 2100 AA Heemstede. Telephone from UK: 00 31 23 529 10 19 Fax from UK: 00 31 23 547 01 19

British Epilepsy Association is a Chapter of IBE representing England and Wales, Epilepsy Association of Scotland is the Chapter representing Scotland and Brainwave (The Irish Epilepsy Association) is the Chapter representing the Republic of Ireland.

Idiopathic Epilepsy The name given to generalised epilepsy which has no known cause. There is no obvious brain damage or disease and the brain seems to be absolutely normal except that there is a tendency towards seizures. Approximately 65% of all epilepsies are idiopathic.

ILAE International League Against Epilepsy - an organisation of doctors which is dedicated towards an ongoing research programme to eventually effect full control of seizures.

The Headquarters of ILAE is: Epilepsie Zentrum Bethel, Mara 1, Maraweg 21, 33617 Bieldefeld, Germany: Telephone from UK: 00 49 521 144 4897 Fax from UK: 00 49 521 144 4637.

Incidence In medical research terms this refers to the number of new diagnoses of a condition occurring in a set population within a given time limit - usually per 100,000 people over a period of one year.

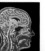

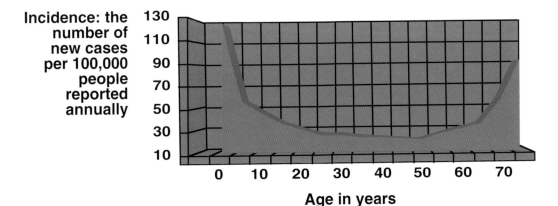

Incidence: the number of new cases per 100,000 people reported annually

Age in years

Various studies have indicated a UK incidence of between 20 -50 per 100,000 population. In the USA the figure is similar. Translated into national populations this means that in the UK as many as 29,000 people each year will be diagnosed as having epilepsy. In the USA the figure will be as many as 125,000.

Applied to a world population the total number of newly diagnosed cases of epilepsy each year is in the region of 2 - 3 million.

Some studies have found a slightly higher incidence in males.

The incidence of epilepsy is at its highest in the age range 0 - 10 years and especially in the first year of life. There is a tail off during adolescence and middle age and it rises again in old age.

Infantile Spasms

Episodes usually begin between the ages of 4 and 7 months. The most frequent seizures are what are best known as 'salaam spasms' when the infant's head very forcefully bends forward whilst at the same time the knees bend and the arms flex. Parents often mistake these events for attacks of wind. When the condition has been recognised an increasingly obvious retardation is noticed. Infantile spasms are a feature of a condition called West Syndrome.

Insurance

People with epilepsy can sometimes find difficulty in getting insurance for life cover, driving or travel. It is always advisable to contact the Epilepsy Associations when seeking cover because invariably they can point the person in the direction of companies which have positive attitudes to those with epilepsy.

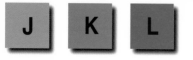

Janz Syndrome This type of epilepsy tends to affect people in the age range 8 - 26 years with the highest proportion being in the 12 - 16 age group.

Myoclonic seizures tend to occur on waking or following a period of sleep deprivation with a jerking of mainly the upper limbs and consciousness is retained throughout.

In 90% of cases people will have generalised tonic-clonic seizures. In about a quarter of cases absence seizures may also occur. There may also be a marked tendency towards photosensitivity in some people.

JEC Joint Epilepsy Council of the UK and Ireland. The organisation represents the major organisations and individuals that work to help people with epilepsy and their carers in the United Kingdom and Ireland. Any of the organisations listed under Epilepsy Associations hold details of the names and addresses of the Officers of the Council.

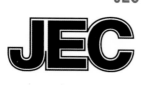

Juvenile Myoclonic Epilepsy See Janz Syndrome.

Ketogenic Diet This is a diet rich in fats and oils which is occasionally prescribed for children with severe epilepsy who have failed to respond to antiepileptic drugs. The main problem with the diet is that it is very unpleasant and the person taking it has to be very dedicated to the regime. Although rarely used in the treatment of epilepsy it has been thought to control seizures in certain cases.

Lamictal® The trade name of the antiepileptic drug lamotrigine.

Lamotrigine The generic name of the antiepileptic drug Lamictal®.

Leisure Activities People with epilepsy can enjoy a full range of leisure activities. For people who experience transitory loss of consciousness or a loss of muscle tone there are some leisure pursuits which are unsuitable. Obvious examples of such activities are mountaineering, deep sea diving or high board diving.

The world of sport presents many opportunities for people with epilepsy to excel and history is littered with the names of famous people who have found great success in theatrical and other artistic activities.

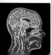

Lennox-Gastaut Syndrome   Children with this syndrome have frequent seizures of different kinds. The onset is most often between the ages of 1 and 3 years and rarely after the age of 7. They usually have complex absence seizures or atonic seizures. Sometimes they can have tonic-clonic seizures.

Children who have Lennox-Gastaut Syndrome may have a series of absences over a very long period of time which makes them behave in a very confused way.

Learning difficulties become apparent at an early age and gradually the retardation accelerates as the child gets older.

Seizures usually continue through adolescence and into adulthood.

Medic Alert   This is a sophisticated effective identification system which can be carried by people who have epilepsy. It gives information about the epilepsy, a special telephone number and a registration number. The information is engraved on the back of an attractive Medic Alert bracelet or a necklace. The jewellery is internationally recognised and full
details can be obtained from the Medic Alert
Foundation,
11 - 13 Clifton Terrace, London N4 3JP.
Tel: 0171 833 3034 .

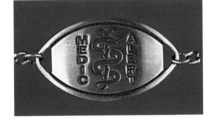

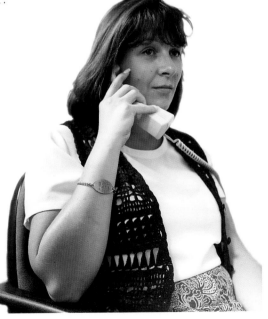

MRI Scanning   This technique produces very clear images of the brain. Many atoms behave like tiny bar magnets. If they are put inside a magnetic field and if the magnetic field is strong enough, these atomic bar magnets can be made to line up and point in the same direction. Radio waves, of a very special frequency, are aimed at the atoms and these echo with their own radio signal. The MRI scanner detects the radio waves and, using computer technology, can build up very detailed pictures.

MRI scans can be used to detect changes in the activity of different regions of the brain. The only known hazard associated with MRI scanning is for people with claustrophobia - there is not a lot of room inside the scanner ! The images can be built up very quickly compared to CT scans.

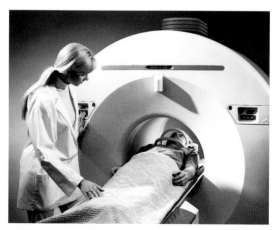

MRI scanner. The patient's head is surrounded by extremely powerful magnets.

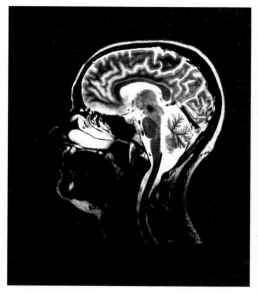

A typical MRI scan, showing the remarkable detail that can be seen.

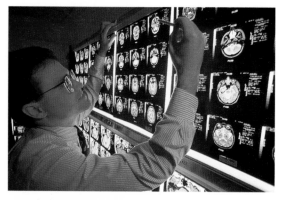

A radiologist inspecting a typical series of MRI scans.

Myoclonic Seizures

"Myo" means muscle and "clonic" means jerk. When myoclonic seizures occur the muscles jerk rather as if the person has had some sort of electric shock. If a person was holding a cup of tea and had a myoclonic seizure the cup and saucer would go flying. It is for this reason that this type of epilepsy has been loosely described as "flying saucer syndrome".

Seizures usually occur shortly after waking or before retiring to bed when the person is tired. There is a loss of consciousness but it is hardly noticeable because the period is so brief. A myoclonic seizure is a type of generalised seizure.

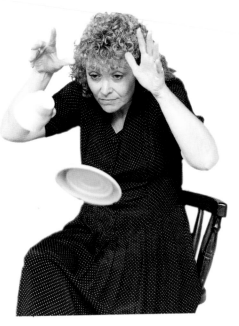

Flying saucer syndrome!

Neurologist

The name given to a doctor who specialises in disorders of the brain and of the nervous system which includes epilepsy. Neurologists work in the hospital service as consultants, advising other physicians on the best form of treatment and management of neurological conditions. It is always advisable to have a diagnosis of epilepsy made, or at least confirmed, by a neurologist.

Neurons

These are the body of cells that make up the brain and the nervous system. They are very small and can only be seen by using a powerful microscope.

Each cell consists of a central part called the body cell, a long tail called the axon and branching off from the axon short tails called dendrites.

Each axon behaves as a wire conducting messages which are passed across an incredible network of neurons via the dendrites.

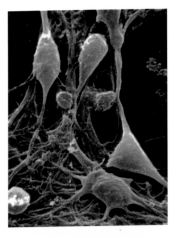

An electron microscope picture of a group of neurons.

The messages are in the form of tiny electrical impulses so it is hardly surprising that if they get out of control seizures occur.

Neurontin®   This is the trade name for the antiepileptic drug gabapentin.

Neurophysiologist   The name given to doctors who specialise in testing the nervous system. Working in hospitals at consultant level they conduct and interpret the results of EEGs of people who are being investigated in relation to epilepsy. Their findings are passed on to neurologists to assist in confirming or denying a clinical diagnosis.

Neuropsychologist   This is a clinical psychologist who specialises in the psychological problems resulting from disorders of the nervous system. Some neuropsychologists work in the hospital service specialising in helping people who cannot come to terms with their epilepsy. A programme of structured sessions is designed to help them with everyday living to improve quality of life. They also play an important part in determining people's suitability for surgical intervention.

Neuroradiologist   The name given to a doctor who specialises in diagnostic techniques to establish problems in the nervous system using conventional X-rays through to CAT Scanners and MRI Scanners. Neuroradiologists work in the hospital service at consultant level in close liaison with other consultants who are treating people with epilepsy.

Neurosurgeon   The name given to a doctor who specialises in the surgery of the nervous system. Neurosurgeons work in the hospital service as consultants. Over recent years there has been an expansion in the work they do to alleviate epileptic seizures and in some specialist units there is a programme of surgical intervention in the treatment of epilepsy.

The Neurosurgeons work closely alongside neurologists, neurophysiologists, neuropsychologists and neuroradiologists in determining those who are suitable to undergo surgery.

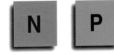

Neurotransmitters — These are naturally occurring chemical substances released from the dendrites of neurons which alter the electrical activity of adjoining neurons.

Nocturnal Seizures — These are seizures which occur during sleeping hours in contrast to diurnal seizures which occur during waking hours.

Non Epileptic Attack Disorder — See Pseudoseizures.

Partial Seizures — Only part of the body is affected by these seizures since the abnormal activity of the brain is localised. There are two types of partial seizures; simple partial seizures and complex partial seizures.

It is possible for a partial seizure to progress to a generalised seizure when the whole brain becomes involved. These generalised seizures are said to be secondarily generalised.

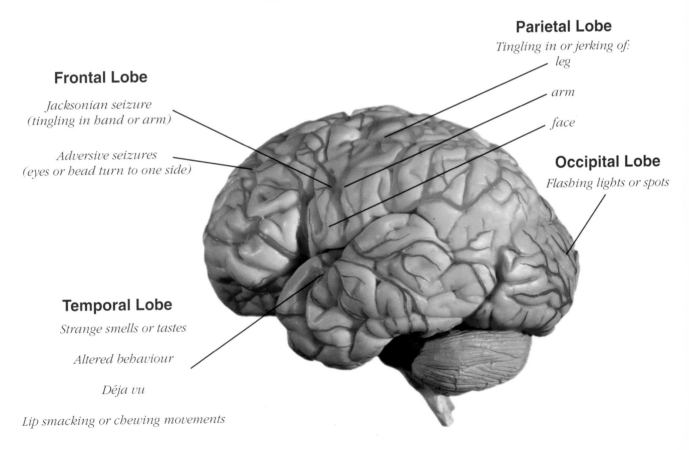

Parietal Lobe
Tingling in or jerking of:
leg
arm
face

Frontal Lobe
Jacksonian seizure (tingling in hand or arm)
Adversive seizures (eyes or head turn to one side)

Occipital Lobe
Flashing lights or spots

Temporal Lobe
Strange smells or tastes
Altered behaviour
Déja vu
Lip smacking or chewing movements

P

Peri-menstrual Seizures Some women have seizures around the time of menstruation. The reason for this is not fully understood. It is possible that a change in hormonal balances provokes seizures.

The likelihood of seizures at this time can sometimes be reduced by taking the drug Frisium® for a few days before the period and on the first day after it starts.

Petit Mal See Absence Seizures.

PET Scanning The letters PET stand for Positron Emission Tomography.

PET scanning provides extremely detailed images of the brain. The patient is injected in the arm with a water solution, which is very slightly radioactive. The energy produced is converted into gamma rays which travel through the brain and are detected by the scanner as they leave the brain. The scanner passes all of this information into a powerful computer, which analyses the patterns detected and builds up an image of the brain. The whole process takes about a minute.

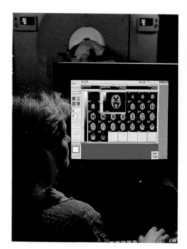

Phenobarbitone This is a long established antiepileptic drug which is used very rarely as a drug of first choice in the treatment of epilepsy.

Phenytoin The generic name of the antiepileptic drug Epanutin®.

Photosensitive Epilepsy Photosensitive epilepsy is the name given to that form of epilepsy in which seizures are provoked by flickering light. Some 2% - 3% of people with epilepsy are affected. Both natural and artificial light sources may precipitate seizures but the most common precipitant appears to be television and the playing of certain computer games.

The first reports of seizures being provoked by watching television were made in the early 1950s. Seizures documented at this stage were said to have been provoked by defective television sets which flickered or whose vertical hold was faulty, causing the picture to roll. Further clinical investigation, however, has indicated the seizures may also be provoked by normally functioning television sets when the viewer is too near the set. Associated factors include the angle from which the set is being viewed,

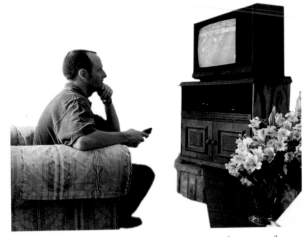

It is important to sit at an adequate distance from the screen. This is too close.

sensitivity to geometric patterns and the effects of tiredness and alcohol.

Various types of seizure may be induced by a flickering light, but a tonic clonic seizure is the most frequent type induced by television, sometimes preceded by myoclonic jerking.

Simple precautions may be taken to avoid having a seizure whilst watching television. The set should always be viewed in a well lit room, from a distance of at least 2 metres, with a small lamp placed on top of the set. The person should avoid approaching the set, adjusting and switching channels, use a remote control unit if possible to adjust settings and channels. If approaching the screen, one eye should be covered. Other conditions precipitating seizures of this type include sunlight reflected off wet surfaces or through leaves, or the flickering effect seen when the subject is moving rapidly past trees or railings illuminated by sunlight shining from the side. Flashing lights such as those used in discos and the flicker of fluorescent lighting may also induce seizures. The wearing of polarised sunglasses out of doors on sunny days is of assistance in removing flickering reflections.

The occurrence of photosensitive seizures has increased since the introduction of VDUs (visual display units) into places of work and schools and also with the popularity of computer games. The VDU, however, is a fact of modern life and it would only be essential to avoid it altogether if advised to do so by the doctor.

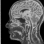

Here are some points to note:

- keep at a distance of 2 - 3 metres away from the television set

- the time spent exposed to the flickering contributes a major part in provoking seizures - ideal VDU time is 15 minutes before taking a 5 minutes break (for television a comparable viewing period is about 30 minutes)

- the contrast must be right for the prevailing environmental lighting and the person's eyes

- sitting at a slight angle to the screen can help

- there are special clip-on screens available to fix to VDUs to cut down the flicker

- word processors do not have the same flicker and flash stimulus as television and computer games, but if they are displayed on personal computers (PCs) then the same rules will apply (although it is usually difficult to sit 2 metres away from the screen) - the only specific guidance is that word processing on a VDU should be avoided when tired.

- covering one eye temporarily or permanently does cut down the effect of flicker but it is best to consult an eye specialist to avoid weakening eyesight

- if the subject wishes to wear shaded lenses an optician should be consulted as many 'polarised' lenses are not always effective and can damage eyesight.

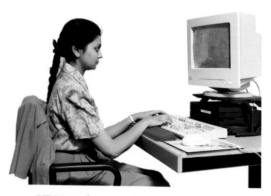

*VDU work inevitably involves viewing a
screen at close quarters.*

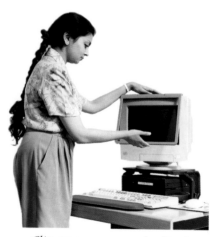

*Clip-on screens can be fitted
to reduce the flicker.*

Precipitating Factors   See Triggers.

Pregnancy and Epilepsy

It is important that women who have epilepsy should plan pregnancies in order to minimise any potential problems which could arise. It is equally important to be aware that 90% of women with epilepsy enjoy normal pregnancies and deliver perfectly healthy babies. Any possible risk of adversities for the other 10% can be minimised by wise preparation and medical advice.

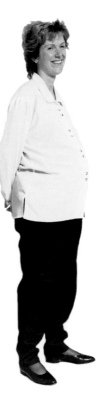

20% of women with epilepsy experience a decrease in seizures during pregnancy, 50% experience no change in seizure pattern and the remaining 30% experience an increase in seizures.

The increased seizure pattern is very often due to the expectant mother reducing levels of antiepileptic medication for fear that the drugs may harm the developing baby. Since the potential to damage the baby is greater as a result of experiencing major convulsive seizures than it is from the drug side effects it is vitally important that the drugs are taken as and when prescribed. It is quite likely that every effort will be made to use as little medication as possible to control seizures. Such issues can be thoroughly discussed with the supervising doctor during the planning time. It is possible that tests to establish drug levels will be performed regularly during the period of pregnancy.

Also during the planning stage it is likely that advice will be given to take vitamins which contain folic acid and to continue taking the preparation during the first three months of pregnancy. The reason for this is that the risk of miscarriage and of foetal malformation is known to be considerably reduced by taking folic acid. Indeed, it is recommended that all pregnant women should take folic acid tablets.

Because the birth of a child can be a stressful and somewhat traumatic event there is a chance that seizures might occur during this period. It is a wise precaution, therefore, that careful consideration be given to hospital confinement rather than home confinement. Close co-operation between the mother, her neurologist and her obstetrician is an essential part of preparation for the actual birth.

Prevalence This, in medical terms, describes the number of people in a population who have a particular condition. It is usually expressed in terms of the number of cases in every 1,000 of the population.

Most studies indicate that the prevalence of epilepsy in the UK is between 4-10 per 1,000 of population. Applied to the whole British population this means that there are as many as half a million people who have epilepsy in the UK.

A recent study in the USA indicated that the prevalence of epilepsy is within the range of 6-10 per 1,000 population. Applied to the whole American population this means that as many as 2.5 million people in the USA have epilepsy.

At best it is reasonable to say that worldwide 20,000,000 people have epilepsy and at worst 60,000,000.

One study established that 2% of all children under the age of 2 years and 7% of children under 7 years were known to have had epileptic seizures.

**Prevalence:
the percentage of
each age group that
has epilepsy at any
given time**

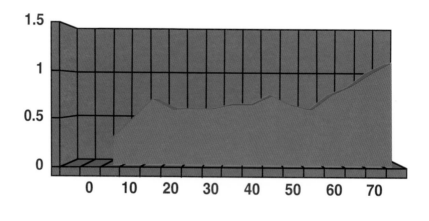

Age in years

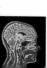

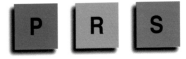

Prognosis   This is the word used to mean the future outlook for a medical condition.

Pseudoseizures   Also known as Non Epileptic Attack Disorder.

Sometimes people simulate seizures, either consciously or unconsciously, giving the false impression that they have epilepsy. Some people with genuine epilepsy may also have pseudoseizures. They are sometimes used for dramatic effect and nearly always happen in the presence of others. Pseudoseizures can be so realistic that an incorrect diagnosis of epilepsy is sometimes made. If this happens, unnecessary antiepileptic drugs can be prescribed.

If it has been established that the episodes being investigated are pseudoseizures the matter is taken up by a neuropsychologist for management and treatment.

Psychomotor Epilepsy   See Complex Partial Seizures or Temporal Lobe Epilepsy.

Research   Throughout the world, there is intensive and costly research taking place into the causes and treatment of epilepsy. Much of this research is funded by pharmaceutical companies to help in developing new antiepileptic drugs. Universities conduct studies into all aspects of the condition and experts regularly present their findings at international medical and scientific meetings.

Rivotril®   The trade name of the antiepileptic drug clonazepam.

Sabril®   The trade name of the antiepileptic drug vigabatrin.

Secondarily Generalised Seizures   It is possible for somebody who has had a partial seizure to then go straight into a generalised seizure. In these cases, the generalised seizure is known as a secondarily generalised seizure, and it is usually atonic, tonic, clonic or tonic-clonic.

Seizure The word 'seizure' is nowadays used to describe an epileptic episode replacing less precise terms such as " fit", "funny turn" or "attack".

When a seizure takes place the brain stops working normally for a short time. In normal circumstances the brain's electrical circuitry is disrupted, the wrong messages are sent and the sufferer cannot control what is happening.

When the disruption occurs in only part of the brain then only one part of the body is affected. In this instance the seizure is classified as being a partial seizure. If, however, the whole brain is affected (and hence the whole body) the seizure is classified as being a generalised seizure.

So varied are the numbers of types of seizures that an international classification of seizures has been drawn up.

Seizure Diary This is a simple chart or a small book for keeping a record of seizures. It is very useful for keeping note of the dates on which seizures occurred and for recording what actually happened. Recording the date presents no problems but often a witness has to be present to get the information about what actually happened.

The recorded information is important in that it helps the neurologist to diagnose the type of epilepsy correctly and so prescribe the correct treatment.

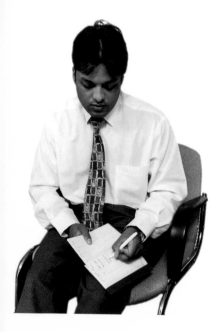

The widespread ownership of portable video cameras has frequently made it possible to record the events of a seizure. The information thus recorded can be given to the neurologist to assist in making the clinical diagnosis.

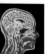

Self-Help Groups See Support Groups.

Simple Partial Seizures These seizures reflect activity in the part of the body controlled by that part of the brain from which the abnormal electrical discharge arises. They can be subdivided into two main types, focal motor seizures and focal sensory seizures. Sometimes simple partial seizures arise only from the temporal lobe of the brain with no other part of the brain being involved. In this type of seizure the person gets an altered sense of perception whilst being completely aware of the surroundings. Such disorientation could show itself as "I feel that I am looking down on myself", "I get a peculiar taste or smell", "I feel as though I have been here before" (deja vu). See also Aura.

There is no alteration or loss of consciousness in a simple partial seizure.

Sodium Valproate The generic name for the antiepileptic drugs Epilim® and Epilim Chrono®.

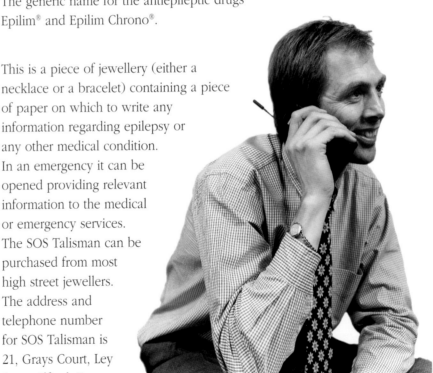

SOS Talisman This is a piece of jewellery (either a necklace or a bracelet) containing a piece of paper on which to write any information regarding epilepsy or any other medical condition. In an emergency it can be opened providing relevant information to the medical or emergency services. The SOS Talisman can be purchased from most high street jewellers. The address and telephone number for SOS Talisman is 21, Grays Court, Ley Street, Ilford, Essex. Tel: 0181 554 5579

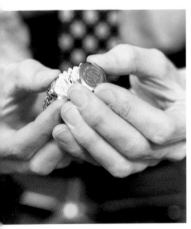

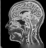

Sport See Leisure Activities.

Status Epilepticus This phrase is used to describe a situation when a seizure is prolonged, or a series of consecutive seizures during which the person does not regain consciousness. Status epilepticus is a medical emergency which requires active treatment by a doctor to stop the seizure.

Stesolid® A trade name for the drug diazepam.

Support Groups The Epilepsy Associations encourage people with epilepsy to meet together and discuss matters of mutual interest. Some groups are formal in structure whilst others are more relaxed, being groups of people who meet socially for as often as they feel it necessary. Both types can be very valuable, especially to people who have been recently diagnosed. Such groups operate throughout the world and are also known as Self-Help Groups.

Surgery For some people whose epilepsy is not controlled with antiepileptic drugs it is possible that an operation may be considered to bring the seizures under control. Not everybody with uncontrolled epilepsy is a suitable candidate for surgery and those who are considered are subjected to a series of tests before a final decision is made as to whether the operation could or should go ahead. The final decision lies with the person who is to have the proposed operation who has to keep in mind all the attendant risks that go along with major surgery and the fact that no guarantees about final outcome can be offered. It is fair to say, however, that there are many people whose quality of life has been improved as a result of an operation to control seizures.

Swimming People with epilepsy should, for their own safety, learn how to swim and enjoy swimming as a leisure activity.

Under controlled conditions the risks from swimming are minimal and under such conditions records of people actually drowning as a result of seizure are very rare.

The social and psychological benefits of swimming for those who have epilepsy are considerable but one must also recognise the risks for people suffering from recurrent seizures because of the unpredictability of the condition. These risks, however, can be minimised not least by choosing a safe place in which to swim.

By far the safest place to go swimming is a well supervised indoor public swimming pool, or a private facility provided it is equally well supervised.

Swimming in outdoor pools, the sea, rivers or in any water below a temperature of 24^0 C (75^0 F) is not recommended.

When using a swimming pool people with epilepsy should inform the pool supervisor of their condition. The supervisor can then keep an eye on the situation, ready to take action if a seizure does occur. Those who are employed at pool sides usually have a life saving qualification but advance notice of a potential hazard is necessary since the person with the epilepsy is not the only one in the pool who has to be supervised.

In any event, it is always best to go swimming with a companion who is a strong swimmer and better still if the companion has life saving qualifications.

The classic sign of the onset of a tonic clonic seizure in the water is a loss of co-ordination in the swimming stroke; the swimmer's sense of direction becomes vague and involuntary head movements may take place.

The first priority is to keep the person's face above water. It is best to approach from behind and, if possible, tow the person in difficulty to shallow water, holding the head until the seizure stops. Medical attention should not be required unless resuscitation is required.

Further detailed advice on the safety of swimming for people with epilepsy can be gained from any of the Epilepsy Associations.

Teenager Clinics As youngsters who have epilepsy mature into adulthood the hospital supervision of treatment transfers from paediatric neurologists to adult neurologists. It is recognised good practice to hold a 'change over clinic' which enables both doctors, along with their respective epilepsy specialist nurses, to discuss future care needs with the young people and their families.

Tegretol® The trade name for the antiepileptic drug carbamazepine.

Tegretol Retard® The trade name for the slow release antiepileptic drug carbamazepine.

Telemetry This is a technique which links a closed circuit television system to an EEG recording system. While the EEG is being recorded a simultaneous video recording is also being made and the information is observed on a split screen VDU, with one half of the screen displaying the EEG trace and the other displaying the person undergoing the test.

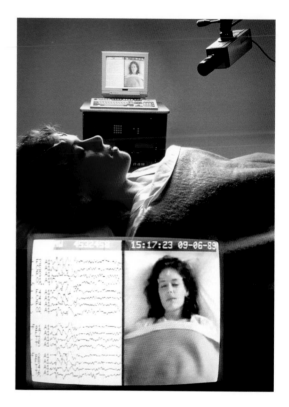

By using telemetry, recordings can be taken over long periods of time and, if required, throughout the night when the patient is sleeping.

Details of what has been happening during the recording period can be played back to establish links between the EEG trace and physical movements.

Temporal Lobe Epilepsy/Seizures See Complex Partial Seizures.

Therapeutic Levels For an antiepileptic drug to work most efficiently, the amount of drug in the bloodstream needs to be at a certain level. Different drugs will have different levels.

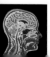

These levels are called the therapeutic levels. If there is any doubt as to whether the levels are correct a simple test can be done whereby a small sample of blood is taken and analysed in a laboratory. If the level is too high or too low the dose can be adjusted accordingly. In practice, most people with epilepsy do not need to have levels checked on a regular basis.

Tiagabine The generic name of the drug Gabatril® which is currently being developed and tested prior to being licensed.

Todd's Paralysis It may happen that a weakness down one side of the body could follow an adversive seizure. This short term weakness is known as Todd's Paralysis.

Tonic Seizures These generalised seizures are quite dramatic. The muscles stiffen and if standing up the person will fall heavily to the floor, often receiving injury to the head. People who are subject to this type of seizure often have to wear protective headwear to avoid constant injury.

Tonic-clonic Seizures These generalised seizures used to be known as 'grand mal' seizures (see convulsion). The seizure starts with a cry and a loss of consciousness with the person falling to the ground. There follows a 'tonic' or stiff phase which leads to a 'clonic' or twitching phase. Finally there may be confusion, often followed by sleep. In addition to the very obvious convulsive movements an observer may see the lips turn blue and if the tongue has been bitten blood may trickle from the mouth with frothy saliva. This may look alarming but is not usually a cause for panic. It is possible, but by no means always the case, that the person could be incontinent or, in rare cases, doubly incontinent.

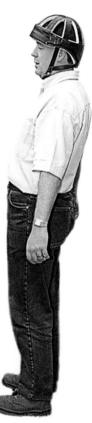

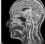

Topamax®   The trade name for the antiepileptic drug topiramate.

Topiramate   The generic name for the antiepileptic drug Topamax®.

Travel   There is no valid reason why people with epilepsy should not enjoy the benefits and pleasure of international travel.   It is wise, however, for them to consider the following points.

Insurance: When taking out medical insurance the small print should be checked as some companies may not offer adequate insurance on the basis that epilepsy promotes greater risk towards accidental injury. The extent of the cover should be checked under the pre-existing medical condition clause (this clause has now been removed by many companies). The Epilepsy Associations will be familiar with companies which do not discriminate against people with epilepsy albeit that they could well seek higher premiums.

Medication Times: Those with epilepsy should be careful to adjust their medication schedules to get a gradual transfer to new time zones. A simple rule is to stick to the usual time interval between doses. It is essential that more than enough medication to last the entire time away from home is taken away. It is also a good idea to carry a written prescription - with the dosage amounts clearly stated - in case of emergency.

For customs purposes medication should be carried in original containers and clearly marked.

General Health: There are certain illnesses which will affect medication including infections and traveller's diarrhoea, both of which cause fluctuations in the levels of antiepileptic drugs in the bloodstream for different reasons. Medical attention should be sought when a person suffers from either of these conditions for more than 24 hours. The use of anti-malarial agents can effect medication and so advice should be sought from a doctor before taking them.

Triggers   All people have a threshold within the brain making them more or less subject to epileptic seizures. Those who have regular seizures have a low threshold and vice versa. This threshold is influenced by many factors and certain events or happenings can lower the threshold and trigger seizures.

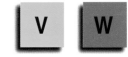

Among the most common triggers are:

- irregular use of medication - neglecting to take prescribed medicine inevitably leads to an increase in the incidence of seizures

- feverish illnesses - rapid rises in body temperature can provoke seizures

- lack of sleep - regular periods of quality sleep are essential in restricting the frequency of seizures

- restricted activity and idleness - it is more likely that a seizure will occur when sitting around with little or nothing to do

- alcohol

- menstruation - see Peri-menstrual epilepsy

- flashing lights - see Photosensitivity

- emotional stress - stress arising from, for example, financial worries or family problems is likely to increase the frequency of seizures.

Valium® A trade name for the drug diazepam.

Vigabatrin® The generic name for the antiepileptic drug Sabril®.

Wada Test This test is done to establish suitability for surgical intervention in the treatment of epilepsy. Under a local anaesthetic a fine tube is inserted into the femoral artery (in the groin) and threaded up the main blood vessel of the body under X-ray guidance, until it lies in the blood vessel supplying half of the brain.

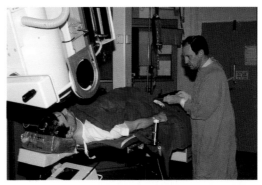

Anaesthetising one half of the brain, via an injection into the femoral artery.

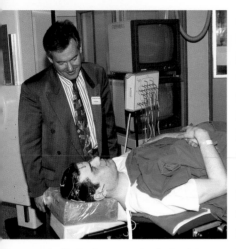

A clinical neuropsychologist questions the patient to test his mental functions.

An anaesthetic drug, Sodium Amytal®, is injected into this blood vessel and puts that side of the brain asleep for a few minutes. The functioning of the other side of the brain is examined with a series of memory tests. The anaesthetic effect does not last long, but while one side of the brain is asleep the other side of the body is temporarily paralysed. When the left side of the brain is anaesthetised there will be a temporary loss of speech. Both sides of the brain are tested.

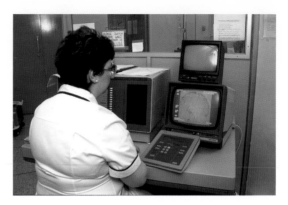

Radiographer acquiring X-rays.

Withdrawal Seizures

Some people who have been free of seizures for many years are tempted to stop taking their medication in the belief that seizures will not recur. Unhappily for them the sudden unsupervised withdrawal of antiepileptic drugs makes it highly likely that seizures will resume.

It is possible, however, for people who have been seizure-free to withdraw from medication, but only under controlled conditions and with close medical supervision. A neurologist will offer the option of a withdrawal programme but will very carefully explain the pros and cons of this course of action.

Zarontin®

The trade name of the antiepileptic drug ethosuximide.